Apple Cider Vinegar Benefits

101 Apple Cider Vinegar Benefits for
Weight Loss, Healthy Skin & Glowing
Hair! Uses for Detoxing, Allergies, Better
Health with Recipes and Cures from
Nature's Remedy

By
Alice Michaels

Apple Cider Vinegar Benefits

By Alice Michaels

Disclaimer

Published by Water Street Press Publishing
2808 Olympia Drive
Grand Prairie, TX 75052

First Printing, 2013

ISBN-13:978-0615910543
ISBN-10:0615910548

Printed in the United States of America

Special Thanks to YOU!

Obtain Your FREE copy of my book "Fat Loss Booster Tips – Get a Boost of Help When You Need it Most"

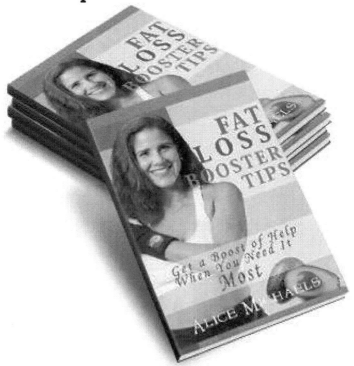

Did you get your FREE copy of my book? Just go to this link on the internet and you'll get all the extras as my gift. ($14.95 value)

Fat Loss Booster Tips – Get a Boost of Help When You Need it Most

http://www.m8u.org/HealthyBonus/

Table of Contents

Millions saw the apple fall, but Newton was the one who asked why.

-Bernard Baruch

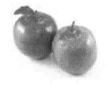

Introduction
An Apple Cider Vinegar Family

Years ago my parents bought a house shaded by a strong and very tall apple tree. The roots grew deep and were watered constantly by a nearby pond.

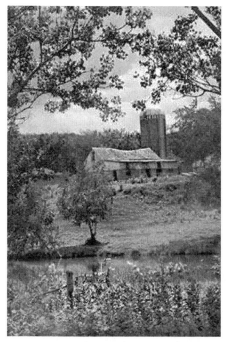

This was the backyard my father would wind into bedtime stories. As the warm and comfortable spring season moved toward summer, the breezes carried a sweet apple blossom fragrance into the kitchen.

All of us had a job coming up that made this part of the year very special for my family. When my mother said the day arrived when I got to help pick apples, I was overjoyed at what this seasonal family gathering time meant. I could grab low hanging apples from the picnic tabletop. My mother would bake pies and give away boxes of apples to friends, who would return later with gallons of apple cider and a few quarts of apple cider vinegar.

I can still feel those warm summer breezes and the happiness and love I spent with my family each summer around the apple tree.

Apple Cider Vinegar has been a staple in many families for generations. The goodness of this vinegar and its benefits go back thousands of years even to the. The real blessing to all of us is that we get many Apple Cider Vinegar benefits that are just as useful today as they were back then.

Alice Michaels

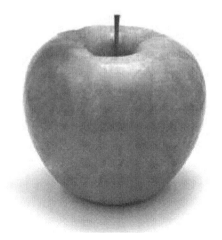

Apple Cider Vinegar Benefits

1) ADHD

Prep Time: 5 min
Application Time: 5 min

Ingredients:
2 T Apple Cider Vinegar
8 oz distilled water

Directions:
A contributing factor that can trigger ADHD is the exposure to toxins. When the digestive system of does not function properly, the bad bacteria increases. The body loses some ability to absorb nutrients. Apple cider vinegar is a good *PRE*-biotic supplement that helps probiotics develop good bacteria balances in the digestive tract. Include up to two tablespoons of Apple cider vinegar three times a day in your daily schedule. Wait at least an hour before taking probiotics. ACV can be either consumed directly or diluted in a glass of filtered water.

2) Age Spots

Prep Time: 10 min
Application Time: 5 to 10 min

Ingredients:
1 OZ Apple Cider Vinegar
Cotton ball
1 oz Strained onion juice

Directions:
Apple cider vinegar can reduce the appearance of age spots, partially reported to do so because it contains sulfur. To reduce age Spots mix Apple cider vinegar with strained onion juice and apply it on the affected area.

Good reports say that you will notice a change within 6 weeks.

3) AIDS Support
Prep Time: 5 min
Application Time: 5 min
Quantity: 3x/day

Ingredients:
3 T Apple Cider Vinegar
8 oz distilled water

Directions:
Improving colon health and balancing constructive and destructive bacteria can increase the time before drugs are needed. 80% of the HIV virus is found in the small and large intestine.* An important fact about HIV is that this virus cannot live or reproduce in an oxygenated environment. Detoxifying the intestines is a helpful method to fight HIV. Apple cider vinegar can assist the gut and intestines in obtaining proper bacteria balances. Taking one tablespoon of Apple Cider Vinegar three times a day can help clean up a toxic colon. Either mix it with water or drink the apple cider vinegar first, but always follow it with water to rinse it off your teeth.

www.naturalnews.com/031914_colon_health_AIDS.html

4) Allergies

Prep Time: 5 min
Application Time: 5 min
Quantity: 1

Ingredients:
1 t. Apple Cider Vinegar
8 oz distilled water

Directions:
Taking a teaspoon of Apple Cider Vinegar can help you fight and prevent various allergies such as sneezing, nose runniness, nose congestion, itchy eyes, red/swollen eyes, itchy ears/throat/lip/mouth etc. Apple cider vinegar has a very strong taste thus; taking it with water is a good idea.

Dilute 1 teaspoon of Apple Cider Vinegar with water, if you cannot bear its strong taste alone.

5) Anxiety
Prep Time: 5 min
Application Time: 5 min
Quantity: 1

Ingredients:
2 t. Apple Cider Vinegar
6 oz distilled water
2 t. Honey

Directions:
If you are suffering from anxiety, try the following recipe to get relief.

Add to a glass of water, two teaspoons of honey and two teaspoons of apple cider vinegar when symptoms appear.

At the onset of the panic attack, take this ACV drink.

There are anecdotal reports that this drink has stopped the progression of panic attacks.

6) Asthma

Prep Time: 5-10 min
Application Time: 30 min

Ingredients:
1 t. Apple Cider Vinegar+ 8 oz distilled water for drinking
½ C Apple Cider Vinegar for soaking cotton pad
Cotton pad

Directions:
Some people vouch that Apple Cider Vinegar relieved them from asthma symptoms. Apple Cider Vinegar is a homemade remedy for asthma and reportedly useful for those who have even used inhalers. Try this method only when you will not be at risk of serious breathing difficulties.

Shake the ACV bottle so that the sediment is evenly spread in the liquid. This sediment has the most healing properties, so it is important to pour a well-shaken ACV into your drink each time.

Drink: Pour a teaspoon of Apple cider vinegar in a glass of water and finish it in sips within half an hour. Do not consume at once.

7) Athletes Foot
Prep Time: 5-10 min
Application Time: 5 to 10 min

Ingredients:
2 oz Apple Cider Vinegar
Cotton pad
Olive Oil (optional)

Directions:
Apple Cider Vinegar is an effective remedy for athlete's foot. Athlete's Foot is a common fungal infection of the skin. Apply it on the affected area with a cotton pad or your fingers. You can also use a spray bottle to spray Apple cider vinegar on the affected area. ACV is a natural disinfectant and anti-fungal, so it will kill some fungus. Be sure to dry your foot completely. Cracked and dry skin can be moisturized with olive oil.

Athletes Foot is easily transmitted to others or back to yourself. Wash socks, shoes and other clothing that has been exposed to your feet, including bedding. Always wear something on your feet to protect them from possible bacteria on floor surfaces.

8) Back pain

Prep Time: 5-10 min
Application Time: 5 to 10 min

Ingredients:
2 oz Apple Cider Vinegar
Cotton pad

Directions:
Not all pain comes from the same causes. Apple cider vinegar is known for its antioxidant and anti- inflammatory properties. Applying it on the back directly can help give relief from some of this type of back pain.

Drinking apple cider vinegar can help relieve back pain that occurs from lactic acid buildup.

-http://drchingchen.com/cider-vinegar-cleanse-for-back-pain-really-yes

9) Bad Breath

Prep Time: 5-10 min
Application Time: 10 sec-10 min

Ingredients:
1 t. Apple Cider Vinegar+ 8 oz distilled water for drinking
½ T ACV+ 1 C distilled water for gargling

Directions:
If you want a natural homemade remedy for bad breath, apple cider vinegar is worth trying. Two common reasons for bad breath is mouth bacteria buildup and improper functioning of the digestive system.

Before using the ACV, be sure to brush and floss your teeth and gums, and scrape your tongue as your dentist has shown you to do. An old dentist joke is "be sure to floss the teeth you want to keep."

Bacteria from food remaining below the gum line and inbetween teeth cause tremendous problems that are often worse than bad breath. After you clean your mouth thoroughly, then take the ACV Drink. Gargle to help eliminate as much odor causing bacteria as possible.

Drink: Take one tablespoon of apple cider vinegar before meal or after meal. You can dilute it with a glass of water to make it taste mild. ACV helps correct digestive bacteria balances that in turn can help stop bad breath. You can also add apple cider vinegar to your food. There are many causes of bad breath. The two mentioned here are some of the most common, but serious conditions can also cause bad breath. Your doctor can help determine causes.

Gargle: Another method is to use apple cider vinegar instead of mouthwash. For this, add a half teaspoon of apple cider vinegar to a cup of water and gargle with this solution for ten seconds instead of using a mouthwash after meal.

10) Bed Sores

Prep Time: 5-10 min
Application Time: 5 to 10 min

Ingredients:
2 oz Apple Cider Vinegar
Cotton pad

Directions:
People who lie on beds or sit in chairs for many hours without rising often suffer from very painful bedsores. Apple cider vinegar can help as a disinfectant in Stage 1 bedsores.

Stage 1 and 2 bedsores can be very painful.

I don't recommend using this on people with Stage 2,3, or 4 bedsores without the approval of your health care professional.

Applying cold Apple Cider Vinegar on the sores can give some relief from the pain. It may also help in decreasing the sore size. However, from my experience, the best thing to manage bedsores is to take pressure off the sore.

11) Bed wetting

Prep Time: 5 min
Application Time: 5 min

Ingredients:
2 Drops Apple Cider Vinegar
6 oz water

Directions:
For children who suffer from bed-wetting, apple cider vinegar can be useful. Some children obtained relief when they were given apple cider Vinegar before going to bed. Just add two little drops of apple cider vinegar in a glass of water and have the child drink this at least an hour before going to bed.

Common bed-wetting often occurs, because different parts of a child's body are growing at different rates. The body requires more fluid, so it will expel more fluid into a bladder that has yet to catch up in size to the greater output by the kidneys.

12) Benign Prostatic Hyperplasia

(Prostatitis)

Prep Time: 5 min
Application Time: as desired

Ingredients:
2 t. Apple Cider Vinegar
8 oz water

Directions:
The Apple Cider Vinegar tonic helps in restoring the body acid and alkaline balance. It improves excretory health reducing prostate problems. Mix 2 teaspoons of apple cider vinegar with a glass of water and sip this in little amounts during the whole day.

13) Bladder infection

Prep Time: 5-7 min
Application Time: 5 min

Ingredients:
2 t. Apple Cider Vinegar
1 t. honey
8 oz water

Directions:
Apple Cider Vinegar and honey is a helpful method to fight bladder infection. Mix the apple cider vinegar with the honey into a glass of water. Drink three times a day.

14) Bleeding

Prep Time: 5 min
Application Time: 5 to 10 min

Ingredients:
½ C Apple Cider Vinegar for soaking cotton pad
Cotton pad

Directions:
Apple cider vinegar is well known for treating wounds and to stop bleeding. ACV has an adrenaline type of effect that is believed to assists in coagulating the blood.

Use a cotton ball soaked in Apple Cider Vinegar and press at the affected area to stop bleeding. Apply it every four hours at the affected area.

15) Body odor

Prep Time: 5-10 min
Application Time: 10 to 15 min

Ingredients:
2 oz Apple Cider Vinegar+ 1 cotton ball for wiping
1/3 C Apple Cider Vinegar+ warm water, enough to soak feet

Directions:
Apple cider vinegar balances the pH level of the body acting effectively against body odor. It eliminates the bacteria that grow and reproduce in sweat and cause body odor.

Wipe: For armpit area, pour undiluted apple cider vinegar on a cotton ball and wipe the area once daily.

Soak: For removing foot odor, soak your feet for 15 minutes in warm water with 1/3 cup of apple cider vinegar in it. This should be repeated every week.

16) Boils

Prep Time: 5 min
Application Time: 5 to 10 min

Ingredients:
½ C Apple cider vinegar
8 oz distilled water
cotton pad

Directions:
Directly applying apple cider vinegar on boils can cause a burning sensation, but it is effective in cleansing the wound. If you cannot tolerate the burning, dilute it with water and then pour on the boils to disinfect them.

17) Bronchitis

Prep Time: 5 min
Application Time: 5 min
Quantity: 1

Ingredients:

1 t. Apple Cider Vinegar
8 oz distilled water
2 T honey

Directions:

Mix 1 tablespoon apple cider vinegar and two teaspoons honey in a glass of warm water. Drink this three times a day, and gargle with it, too. Gargling with ACV can kill some bacteria in the mouth. Drinking ACV can reduce phlegm associated with congestion.

18) Free radicals

Prep Time: 5 min
Application Time: 5 min

Ingredients:
2 T Apple Cider Vinegar +8 oz distilled water

Directions:
Beta-carotene present in apple cider vinegar possesses anti-oxidant properties, helping to counteract the damage caused by free radicals. Reducing free radicals gives a boost to the immune system and works to prevent metabolic disorders. Include two tablespoonfuls of apple cider vinegar mixed in a glass of water three times a day.

19) Bruising

Prep Time: 5 min
Application Time: 5-10

Ingredients:
½ C Apple Cider Vinegar for soaking cotton pad
Cotton pad

Directions:
The anti-inflammatory properties of apple cider vinegar can shrink capillaries and reduce swelling and redness of a bruise. Pour apple cider vinegar on a cotton pad and apply to the bruise. Appearance change within one hour is common and the bruise will vanish a little faster than normal.

20) Bunions

Prep Time: 5-10 min
Application Time: 20 to 25 min

Ingredients:
2 C Apple cider vinegar+ 4 C warm water
Olive oil

Directions:
To treat bunions, mix two cups of apple cider vinegar with four cups of warm water. Soak your feet in this for about 20-25 minutes. After 15 minutes of soaking, massage area gently with olive oil.

21) Burns

Prep Time: 5 min
Application Time: 5 to 10 min
Quantity: 1

Ingredients:
1 C Apple cider vinegar
Washcloth

Directions:
Minor burns can be treated with apple cider vinegar. Soak a washcloth in apple cider vinegar and apply to the burn. It can cause a slight stinging or itchy effect. Notice a relief from pain.

22) Bursitis

Prep Time: 5 min
Application Time: 5 min
Quantity: 1

Ingredients:
2 T Apple cider vinegar
8 oz water

Directions:
To get relief from bursitis it is essential to balance the fluid volume in the body. Drinking two tablespoons of Apple Cider Vinegar with water each day is one of the oldest remedies that can restore alkalinity to help maintain the balance necessary for treating bursitis. Be sure to rest the area of inflammation. Adding external ice packs or alternating with ice packs and heat is helpful, too.

23) Cancer Support

Prep Time: 5 min
Application Time: 5 min
Quantity: 1

Ingredients:
2 T Apple cider vinegar
8 oz water

Directions:
http://www.webmd.com/diet/apple-cider-vinegar?page=2
According to WebMd, there are studies with promising revelations regarding cancer and treatment with vinegar.

"A few laboratory studies have found that vinegar may be able to kill cancer cells or slow their growth. Observational studies of people have been confusing. One found that eating vinegar was associated with a decreased risk of esophageal cancer. Another associated it with an increased risk of bladder cancer."

The free radicals formed in our bodies are due to oxidation that can cause various types of cancers.

Anti-oxidants help keep a check on free radicals. Beta- carotene present in Apple Cider Vinegar is a very powerful anti-oxidant.

It helps in neutralizing the free radicals. However, it cannot cure cancer. Take Apple Cider Vinegar diluted in a glass of water three times a day.

24) Candidiasis

Prep Time: 5 min
Application Time: 5 min
Quantity: 1

Ingredients:
2 T Apple cider vinegar
8 oz lukewarm water

Directions:
Candida is a yeast infection that is easily created and destroyed through diet changes. A cheap remedy for candida is apple cider vinegar that is rich in nutrients and natural enzymes. It reduces the yeast causing candida. Drink two tablespoons of apple cider vinegar with a glass of lukewarm water three times a day until the symptoms disappear completely.

25) Canker sores

Prep Time: 5-7 min
Application Time: 5 min
Quantity: 1

Ingredients:
2 T Apple cider vinegar
1 T calcium- magnesium powder
4 oz warm water
4 oz cold water

Directions:
To help get rid of canker sores, add two tablespoons of apple cider vinegar and a tablespoon of calcium-magnesium powder to 4 ounces of warm water. Fill the rest of glass with cold water and sip this mixture over the sore.

26) Carbuncles

Prep Time: 5-10 min
Application Time: as desired

Ingredients:
1 C apple cider vinegar
Pieces of stale bread
Waterproof bandage

Directions:
For healing carbuncles, dip a piece of stale bread in Apple Cider Vinegar and apply it on the carbuncle. Cover it with waterproof bandage and leave overnight. Remove the bread in the morning and reapply with another piece for use during the day. Continue this process until the carbuncle has disappeared.

27) Carpal Tunnel Syndrome

Prep Time: 5 min
Application Time: 5 min

Ingredients:
1 T Apple cider vinegar
8 oz distilled water

Directions:
Carpal tunnel syndrome can be exacerbated by inflammation. Apple Cider Vinegar has anti-oxidants that help lessen the painful effects of this syndrome when inflammation is the primary cause of pain. Apple Cider Vinegar is much cheaper than anti-inflammation medicines. Drink a tablespoon of Apple Cider Vinegar in a glass of water up to three times a day to help reduce carpal tunnel syndrome.

28) Cataracts

Prep Time: 5- 10 min
Application Time: 10 to 14 min
Quantity: 1 use per eye

Ingredients:
2/3 t apple cider vinegar
4 oz distilled water
eye dropper or eyewash cup

Directions:
Apple Cider Vinegar can be an effective remedy for cataracts in both human and animals when the cause is a cloudy protein film obscuring vision. Patricia Bragg's recommends 1/3 t of Bragg's organic apple cider vinegar diluted with 4 oz of distilled water. Hold eyes closed a few minutes after adding a few diluted drops or using the eyewash cup. Use up to 3 times each day.

29) Cellulite

Prep Time: 5-10 min
Application Time: 10 to 20 min

Ingredients:
1 T Apple Cider Vinegar + 8oz distilled water for drinking
3 T Apple Cider Vinegar + 1 T massage oil

Directions:
For temporary smoothing of cellulite:

Drink: Mix two tablespoons of Apple Cider Vinegar in a glass of water and drink it empty stomach, every morning.

Massage: Another method is to mix three parts of Apple Cider Vinegar with one part of any massage oil and massage the affected area with this once daily.

Add regular exercise and an improved diet to remove cellulite permanently.

30) Chicken Pox

Prep Time: 5 min
Application Time: as desired

Ingredients:
1 C Apple cider vinegar
1 Bucket water

Directions:

Apple Cider Vinegar is very soothing for chicken pox. Mix one cup of Apple Cider Vinegar in a bucket of water to get relief from itching, if you have chicken pox. It also helps in controlling the infection.

31) Chiggers

Prep Time: 5 min
Application Time: 10 to 15 min

Ingredients:
1 oz apple cider vinegar
1 oz distilled water
spray bottle

Directions:
Mix equal amounts of Apple Cider Vinegar and water and apply on the area affected by chigger bite to help relieve pain and itching.

Preventative:
Before entering known areas that may harbor chiggers, spray this mixture on your body to repel them naturally. Adjust the ACV strength closer to full strength in order to find the strength that works for you. Full strength ACV has occasionally burned highly sensitive skin.

32) Chronic Fatigue

Prep Time: 5 min
Application Time: 5 min

Ingredients:
1 C honey
3 T apple cider vinegar

Directions:
For chronic fatigue, mix 1 cup of honey and 3 tablespoons of apple cider vinegar. Keep this mixture near your bed. Take two tablespoons of this half an hour before going to bed. If you wake up during the night, take two more tablespoons of this mixture.

33) Cirrhosis Support

Prep Time: 5 min
Application Time: 5 min

Ingredients:
1 T apple cider vinegar
8 oz distilled water

Directions:
ACV can detoxify the body and work to remove the accumulated fat around the liver. It can break down fat over time and help increase a healthy functioning liver. Drink one tablespoon of Apple Cider Vinegar consumed either directly or with a glass of water three times a day to reduce liver inflammation and irritation.

34) Cold Sores

Prep Time: 5-7 min
Application Time: 5 to 10 min

Ingredients:
1 oz apple cider vinegar
1 T lemon juice

Directions:
Mix Apple Cider Vinegar with lemon juice and apply it on the sores. Putting Apple Cider Vinegar on an open sore will cause a lot of burning, so it is better to apply it before the sore opens up. Right method to apply it is to pour it on a cotton ball and place it on the sore for few minutes.

35) Cold and flu

Prep Time: 10-15 min
Application Time: 20 to 25 min

Ingredients:

1 T apple cider vinegar+8 oz water (drinking)
1 C apple cider vinegar+ Brown paper+ 50 g pepper (applying)

Directions:

Apple Cider Vinegar helps in balancing the pH level of the body and can prevent or reduce the harshness of colds and the flu.

Drink: Take Apple Cider Vinegar three times a day diluted in water.

Apply: Another remedy goes like this- Dampen a brown paper with Apple Cider Vinegar and place pepper at one side of the paper. Tie this paper on the chest for 20-25 minutes with the pepper on the side touching your chest. This gives relief in cold and flu.

36) Colitis

Prep Time: 5 min
Application Time: 5 min

Ingredients:
2 T apple cider vinegar
1 T honey
8 oz distilled water

Directions:
The Apple Cider Vinegar and honey treatment has been found very effective in treating colitis. Two tablespoons of Apple Cider Vinegar with one tablespoon of honey mixed in a glass of water can offer some relief against colitis. Take up to three times a day.

37) Colon Cancer Support

Prep Time: 5 min
Application Time: 5 min

Ingredients:
2 T apple cider vinegar
8 oz distilled water

Directions:
Apples have positive effects on colon health. Consumption of Apple Cider Vinegar can increase fatty acid that is produced in the lower colon. Apple Cider Vinegar contains some insoluble fibers that encourage bowel movements. However, it will not cure the cancer. Two tablespoons of Apple Cider Vinegar should be diluted in a glass of water and consumed three times a day to help normalize bowel movements.

38) Conjunctivitis

Prep Time: 5-7 min
Application Time: 10- 15 sec
Quantity: 1 use per eye

Ingredients:
Apple Cider Vinegar as needed
4 T distilled water
2 cotton balls

Directions:
People suffering from conjunctivitis can get relief by using an apple cider vinegar wash, drops and cotton ball applications.   Apple Cider Vinegar cannot be directly poured into the eyes.   Mix a teaspoon of it with four teaspoon of filtered water. Dampen a sterilize cotton ball with this solution and wipe the affected eyes two-three times a day. Always use a new cotton ball for each application.

Patricia Bragg's recommends 1/3 t of Bragg's organic apple cider vinegar diluted with 4 oz of distilled water. Hold eyes closed a few minutes after adding a few diluted drops or using the eyewash cup. Use up to 3 times each day.

39) Constipation

Prep Time: 5 min
Application Time: 5 min

1 T apple cider vinegar
8 oz distilled water

Directions:
Soluble fiber in Apple Cider Vinegar encourages regular bowel movements. Balancing the pH of the body also helps to normalize water content of the bowels that lead to normal movements.

Drink a tablespoon of Apple Cider Vinegar three times each day to help reduce constipation by producing essential digestive acids in the body, increasing soluble fiber and proper elimination.

There are many causes of constipation from medications to disease, but the most common cause is from diets that do not contain enough fibrous fruits and vegetables.

40) Corns

Prep Time: 6-10 min
Application Time: 10 to 20 min

Ingredients:
1 oz Apple Cider Vinegar
1 oz tea tree oil
2 cotton balls
pumice stone

Directions:
This is a very less known, but an effective treatment for corns. Soak a cotton ball in Apple Cider Vinegar and keep it on the corn for 3-5 minutes. Then dry the area by gently patting it with a soft dry cloth. When the area is completely dry, soak another cotton ball in tea tree oil and again apply it to the area for 3-5 minutes. Repeat this for two to three days until you see the corn peeling up, then, smoothen the area with a pumice stone.

41) Cough

Prep Time: 5-8 min
Application Time: 5 min
Quantity: 1

Ingredients:
2 t. Apple Cider Vinegar
8 oz distilled water
2 T honey

Directions:
The simple of Simple coughs can be treated effectively with the Apple Cider Vinegar recipe. Mix two teaspoons of Apple Cider Vinegar and two teaspoons of honey in a glass of water. Gargle and drink before meals. Keep this near your bed during the night so to sip when coughing may keep you awake.

42) Cuts

Prep Time: 5 min
Application Time: 10 to 14 min

Ingredients:
1 oz Apple Cider Vinegar
Cotton balls

Directions:
Minor cuts can be treated with apple cider vinegar. To stop bleeding, soak a cotton ball in Apple Cider Vinegar and keep it on the affected area. Apply it regularly on the affected area two-three times a day to help heal the cut and minimize scarring.

43) Dandruff

Prep Time: 5-10 min
Application Time: half an hour

Ingredients:
½ C Apple Cider Vinegar
1 cotton ball

Directions:
The main ingredient of Apple Cider Vinegar is acetic acid and can help you get rid of the dandruff on the scalp. It kills bacteria on the scalp, reduces dandruff and leaves your hair soft and shiny. It is useful in almost every problem related with hair and scalp such as some baldness, itching and dermatitis. Apply Apple Cider Vinegar to the scalp about half an hour before bath and then rinse it off.

44) Depression

Prep Time: 5 min
Application Time: 5 min
Quantity: 1

Ingredients:
1 T apple cider vinegar
8 oz distilled water

Directions:
Improper functioning of liver, digestive system can trigger depression. Apple Cider Vinegar can detoxify the body, maintain the alkalinity of body, and encourage healthy functioning of liver and kidneys. A tablespoon of Apple Cider Vinegar three times a day can help in fighting depression. You can also mix one tablespoons of Apple Cider Vinegar with a glass of water if you don't like its strong taste.

45) Dermatitis

Prep Time: 7- 10 min
Application Time: 6 to 10 min

Ingredients:
1/3 C Apple Cider Vinegar
1/3 C distilled water
1 T tea tree oil
1 sachet Head & Shoulders shampoo

Directions:
Mix 1/3 cup of organic Apple Cider Vinegar with 1/3 cup of water, small amount of Head and Shoulders shampoo and tea tree oil. Apply this mixture on scalp, face and all other affected areas. Keep for some minutes and then rinse off. Repeat this three times a week. Organic Apple Cider Vinegar has acetic acid that fights infection and kills bacteria. Tea tree oil is a good natural antibacterial and antifungal.

46) Diabetes

Prep Time: 5 min
Application Time: 5 min

Ingredients:
2 T apple cider vinegar
8 oz distilled water

Directions:
Apple Cider Vinegar can improve stability among those who suffer from Type II diabetes.

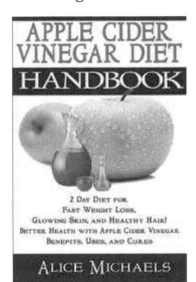

Dietary fiber in Apple Cider Vinegar controls blood sugar levels by slowing the transport of dietary sugars from the intestines into the blood system. Two tablespoons of ACV can taken three times a day directly or diluted in a glass of water.

Hunger cravings are also reduced, so maintaining a better diet becomes easier.

Apple Cider Vinegar DIET Handbook

by Alice Michaels

47) Diaper rash

Prep Time: 5-7 min
Application Time: 3 to 6 min

Ingredients:
1 t. Apple Cider Vinegar
½ C distilled water
1 cotton ball

Directions:
Diluted Apple Cider Vinegar can be used to heal diaper rash. Mix about a teaspoon of Apple Cider Vinegar with a half cup of water. Apply this on the rash with a soft cotton ball or cloth. It has anti-bacterial properties that heals the rash. Make sure that the rash is not too severe as it can be stingy for your baby.

48) Diarrhea

Prep Time: 5 min
Application Time: 5 min

Ingredients:
1 t. apple cider vinegar
8 oz distilled water

Directions:
The pectin in Apple Cider Vinegar is incredible in treating diarrhea as the soluble fiber swells up and forms bulk. It also fights the bacteria that cause diarrhea. The pectin is transformed into a coating that protects the irritated lining of the colon. Apple Cider Vinegar also helps in digestion, bowel movements and elimination. Due to its healing properties, you can get relief from diarrhea easily. One teaspoon of Apple Cider Vinegar should be taken with a glass of water before and between meals. In total, it should be six glasses in a day.

49) Diverticulitis

Prep Time: 5 min
Application Time: 5 min

Ingredients:
1 t. apple cider vinegar
8 oz distilled water

Directions:
Diverticulitis is a digestive disease found in the large intestine. There are diverticula (pouches) outside the colon. If one of these diverticula becomes inflamed, it leads to Diverticulitis. It can be treated by taking a teaspoon of Apple Cider Vinegar with a glass of water three times a day. Apple Cider Vinegar keeps the digestive track healthy.

50) Dizziness

Prep Time: 5- 10 min
Application Time: 5 min
Quantity: 1

Ingredients:
1 t. Apple Cider Vinegar
2 T honey
8 oz distilled hot or cold water

Directions:
Dizziness causes are varied from temperature changes to simple nutritional deficiencies to more severe causes such as debilitating and dangerous diseases. For severe causes of dizziness, the ACV drink may be supportive, but should not be used as a primary assist.

One teaspoon of apple cider vinegar with two teaspoons of honey in a glass of hot or cold water can help control dizziness, especially when blood sugar is low. Taken this three times a day. Although this may not give instant results, in time there can be a decrease in the intensity of dizziness. Do not take in case of diabetes..

51) Ear Infections

Prep Time: 5-10 min
Application Time: 10 to 14 min
Quantity: 1 use each ear

Ingredients:

1 oz Apple Cider Vinegar
1 oz distilled water
2 cotton balls

Directions:

Fungal infections in the ear can obtain relief naturally with apple cider vinegar. Mix Apple Cider Vinegar and distilled water in equal amounts and soak a cotton ball in it. Turn the head so the ear to treat is upward. Place the soaked cotton ball gently at the entrance to the ear and leave for 5-7 minutes. Remove the cotton ball and dry the ear. Repeat this twice daily until the infection is gone.

52) Eczema

Ingredients:
1 T Apple Cider Vinegar+ 8oz distilled water for drinking
2 C Apple cider vinegar+ enough water to bath.

Directions:
Apple Cider Vinegar is effective at relieving some symptoms of eczema.   Apple Cider Vinegar also contains the powerful anti-oxidant, Beta- carotene that helps in cell renewal and ensures good skin health. Apple Cider Vinegar also has anti- fungal and anti-bacterial properties that relieves itchiness and inflammation.

Drink: 1 tablespoon of Apple Cider Vinegar in a glass of water three times a day, half an hour before meals to combat Eczema. You can also add a spoonful of honey to make it taste better.

Bath: Mix 2 cups of Apple Cider Vinegar with a bucket of lukewarm water and have a bath with this three times a week. For instant relief from itchiness and dryness, dilute 1 tablespoon of Apple Cider Vinegar with a cup of water and apply on the affected area.

53) Edema

Prep Time: 5 min
Application Time: 5 min

Ingredients:
1 oz Apple Cider Vinegar
1 oz distilled water
2 cotton balls

Directions:
Edema can be treated with help of Apple Cider Vinegar as it removes extra fluids from the body. It is also incredible in reducing the swelling that comes with edema. Consume 1 tablespoon of Apple Cider Vinegar mixed in a glass of filtered water, up to three times daily. You can also wrap the place where the swelling appears to help reduce inflammation and pain. Mix equal amounts of Apple Cider Vinegar and water and soak a large cotton ball in it. Let the cotton ball rest at the affected place for 5 minutes and then remove. Try this 2-3 times daily.

54) Endurance

Prep Time: 10 min
Application Time: 5 min
Quantity: 1

Ingredients:
1 T Apple Cider Vinegar
8 oz distilled water

Directions:
Lactic acid accumulates in muscles during exercise causing fatigue. Give yourself a boost during an intense workout with a shot of apple cider vinegar. Follow it with extra water to keep the acid level low on your teeth and gums. Or after workouts, mix one tablespoon of Apple Cider Vinegar in a glass of water and consume after work-outs. Take three times a day for overall health.

55) Epilepsy

Prep Time: 5 min
Application Time: 5 min

Ingredients:
1 T apple cider vinegar
8 oz distilled water

Directions:

Add a tablespoon of Apple Cider Vinegar three times a day in your schedule and get a relief in epilepsy. Apple Cider Vinegar can be taken directly or diluted in a glass of water because its taste is very sour and some people can't consume it alone.

56) Erectile Dysfunction

Prep Time: 5 min
Application Time: 5 min

Ingredients:
1 T apple cider vinegar
8 oz distilled water

Directions:
Erectile dysfunction also called ED is a disease in which a man is incapable of maintaining erections for sexual intercourse. This becomes more common as men age into their 50's, but some men suffer from this disease when they are in their 20's. Erectile dysfunction can be treated by adding a spoonful of Apple Cider Vinegar three times a day in your diet. You can mix it with a glass of water to make it taste mild.

57) Esophageal Cancer Support

Prep Time: 5 min
Application Time: 5 min

Ingredients:
1 T apple cider vinegar
8 oz distilled water

Directions:
See CANCER

58) Fainting

Prep Time: 5-10 min
Application Time: 5-10 min

Ingredients:

2 T Apple Cider Vinegar+2 T honey+8 oz water (prevention)

3 oz Apple Cider Vinegar+ handkerchief (relief)

Directions:

The honey and Apple Cider Vinegar is a very popular treatment for fainting.

Drink for dizziness: 2 T of apple cider vinegar, 2 T of honey mixed in a glass of water.

Apply after fainting: Soak a handkerchief or cloth in apple cider vinegar and place under the nose.

59) Fibromyalgia

Prep Time: 5 min
Application Time: 5 min

Ingredients:
2 T apple cider vinegar
8 oz distilled water

Directions:
Apple cider vinegar stimulates digestion and especially the pancreas. The apple cider vinegar tonic helps to restore the body acid and alkaline balance. It is also very effective to help relive joint pains associated with some forms of arthritis.

Drink: Mix 2 tablespoons of apple cider vinegar to 8 oz. of water. Drink up to 3 times a day.

60) Flatulence

Prep Time: 10 min
Application Time: 5 min

Ingredients:
2 T apple cider vinegar
8 oz lukewarm distilled water

Directions:
Primary causes of 'flatulence' are indigestion and bacteria imbalance. Apple cider vinegar can help restore good:bad bacteria balance and improve body alkalinity.

Drink: 2 tablespoons of apple cider vinegar in a glass of lukewarm water up to three times a day before meals

61) Food Poisoning

Prep Time: 5 min
Application Time: 5 min

Ingredients:
1 T apple cider vinegar
8 oz distilled water

Directions:
Apple Cider Vinegar is known for its alkaline properties. When consumed, it soothes the intestinal lining, improves digestion and kills harmful bacteria.

As a first aide to control food poisoning:
Drink a tablespoon of apple cider vinegar diluted in a glass of distilled water three times a day

Some food poisonings are deadly. Minor food poisoning can often be eliminated with ACV, but serious food poisoning requires a visit to your doctor or the emergency room.

62) Strengthen Bones

Prep Time: 5 min
Application Time: 5 min

Ingredients:
2 T apple cider vinegar
8 oz distilled water

Directions:
Apple cider vinegar is rich in minerals like manganese, calcium, magnesium, silicon and iron. All these help to develop and strengthen bones. Include apple cider vinegar shots in your schedule for good bone health

Drink: take two tablespoons each of apple cider vinegar and honey, and mix it in a glass of water. Drink up to three times a day.

63) Fungal Infections

Prep Time: 7-10 min
Application Time: 5-10 min

Ingredients:

1 C Apple Cider Vinegar+ enough water (feet, nails)

1 oz Apple Cider Vinegar+ cotton ball (for skin adults)

1 oz Apple Cider Vinegar+1 C water+ cotton ball (children)

Directions:

Fungal infections in the body can be reduced or eliminated by using apple cider vinegar. Fungal infections can indicate a systemic problem. Drink 2T of ACV in water 3 times each day. For foot, toe or nail fungus, mix 1 cup of apple cider vinegar in one-third bucket of water. Soak your feet/nails for 5 minutes. Repeat each day until the infection is gone.

If the infection is on skin, apply apple cider vinegar directly on the affected area with a sterilized cotton ball. Those who have sensitive skin can dilute ACV with equal parts of water before direct application

64) Gallbladder Disorders

Prep Time: 5 min
Application Time: 5 min

Ingredients:
2 T apple cider vinegar
8 oz distilled water

Directions:
Apple cider vinegar has been found to dissolve or soften some gallstones, and assist in helping other gallbladder disorders. It is also said to reduce the size of the gallbladder stones.

~http://aroundmyhome.blogspot.com/2009/03/what-i-did-to-get-rid-of-my-gallstones.html.

Two tablespoons of apple cider vinegar mixed with a glass of water can be taken up to three times a day. Restricting fat in the diet can minimize painful attacks. Just how long and how much ACV it will take to reduce or eliminate the stones is unknown, because not all stones are the same

65) General Ailments

Prep Time: 5-15 min
Application Time: 5 to 154 min

Ingredients:

2 T Apple Cider Vinegar+ 8 oz distilled water (drinking)

1 C Apple Cider Vinegar+ enough water (bathing)

1 C Apple Cider Vinegar+ enough water for soaking

1 oz apple cider vinegar+1 oz water+ cotton ball (treating sores, acne etc.)

2 T Apple Cider Vinegar+ 8 oz water (gargling)

Directions:

Apple Cider Vinegar can be used to treat many ailments. For generations it has been considered a tonic used to maintain overall health. Some of the general ailments it can give relief in are as below-

Sinus infections and sore throats
Reduce gum/teeth infection.
High cholesterol
Acne
Food poisoning
Allergies
Muscle fatigue after exercise
Arthritis and gout
Bladder stones and urinary tract infections
Strengthen the immune system
Increase stamina
Promote weight loss

Improve digestion

Drink: Dilute Two tablespoons of apple cider vinegar with a glass of filtered water and consume three times a day for overall health.

Skin disorders: Dilute a cup of apple cider vinegar in a bucket of warm water and take bath three times in a week to prevent skin disorders and allergies.

Soak: Soak hand/feet/nails in a cup of Apple Cider Vinegar mixed with water to treat gout, fungal infection, nail infection etc. Soak the affected area for 5 minutes two times daily.

Burn/sores/acne etc.: Apply it mixed with equal amount of water on affected areas such as sores, acne, sunburn, minor burn etc. It can be applied on the affected area with a cotton ball for 3-5 minutes two times daily.

Gargle: Mix two tablespoons of Apple Cider Vinegar in a glass of water and use as a mouthwash or gargle to get relief in mouth and throat infection.

66) Gout

Prep Time: 5 min
Application Time: 10 to 14 min

Ingredients:
1 C Apple Cider Vinegar
Enough water to soak

Directions:
Gout can be caused by excess uric acid in the body. Gout is "a medical condition usually characterized by recurrent attacks of acute inflammatory arthritis—a red, tender, hot, swollen joint."[1] Gout is also considered a disease by diet.

Avoid these foods: [2]
Fish and other foods high in purine
1. Alcohol, especially beer
2. Coffee, a diuretic that increases the uric acid concentration from blood to joints
3. Organ meats, particularly high in purine
4. Fatty fried foods
5. Beef especially, contains highest amount of purine
6. Fructose sweetened fruit drinks and sodas
7. Sauces, high fat
8. Shellfish

Soak: Mix a cup of apple cider vinegar in water and immerse your feet in it for 5 minutes. Remove and pat dry. Repeat the process twice daily until the gout improves or disappears

Drink: Take 2 T of apple cider vinegar with 8 oz of water up to 3x daily.

[1] HTTP://EN.WIKIPEDIA.ORG/WIKI/GOUT
[2] http://www.activebeat.co/diet-nutrition/10-trigger-foods-for-gout/

67) Gum Disease

Prep Time: 5 min
Application Time: 5 to 10 min

Ingredients:
1 oz Apple Cider Vinegar (direct applying)
2 T Apple Cider Vinegar+ 8 oz water (gargling)

Directions:
Apple cider vinegar is helpful in reducing symptoms of gum diseases, such as bad breath, swollen gums, bleeding of the gums, pain and sensitivity around the gums. ACV has anti- bacterial and anti-fungal properties to combat gum diseases

Apple cider vinegar can help keep gums healthy, but it cannot replace good oral hygiene. Brushing and flossing properly remove food that breeds bacteria. Follow your dentist's recommendations with brushing and flossing, then gargle, and apply ACV.

Gargle: Mix two tablespoons of Apple Cider Vinegar in a glass of water and gargle 2-3 times each day.

Apply: Apple Cider Vinegar can also be applied directly to the gums for instant relief. It has both healing and soothing properties. Using apple cider vinegar also prevents some gum diseases by reducing harmful bacteria growth.

68) Hair Loss

Prep Time: 10 min
Application Time: 30 min

Ingredients:
3-4 T Apple Cider Vinegar
4 oz water
sprig of rosemary or twist of lemon

Directions:
Apple cider vinegar can help keep your scalp and hair healthy.

Good blood circulation is needed for healthy and strong hair. Apple cider vinegar helps increase the circulation of blood into the hair roots thereby strengthening the roots and promoting growth.

Due to use of continuous cosmetic products, the pH balance of hair is disturbed leading to hair loss. Apple cider vinegar maintains the pH level to create an optimum environment for hair growth..

Apple cider vinegar has anti-fungal and anti-bacterial properties that help keep bacteria, dandruff and other scalp problems from spreading that also can cause hair fallout.

Use apple cider vinegar to stop hair fallout and gain healthy and shiny hair:

1. Mix 3-4 tablespoons of apple cider vinegar with half glass of water.
2. Add the rosemary or lemon and shake well.
3. Massage into scalp and hair for 30 minutes before bathing.
4. Then rinse out with cold water

69) Hangover

Ingredients:
2 T apple cider vinegar
8 oz distilled water

Directions:
Large quantities of alcohol leave toxins in our bodies, especially in the liver. Apple cider vinegar is believed to help eliminate these toxins.

Many essential minerals are depleted in our bodies due to excess alcohol consumption.

Apple cider vinegar can replace some potassium, calcium, magnesium, sodium and iron. Two tablespoons of ACV mixed with a glass of water can help minimize the hangover.

Plan ahead: The day before and day of indulging, drink up to 3 ACV drinks each day.
Day After: Drink up to 3 ACV drinks again.

70) Hay-Fever

Prep Time: 5-7 min
Application Time: 5 min

Ingredients:
2 T apple cider vinegar
2 T honey
8 oz distilled water

Directions:

For some people the honey and apple cider vinegar recipe is incredible in treating Hay fever. Expect results within a few days.

Hay fever signs and symptoms usually start immediately after you're exposed to a specific allergy-causing substance (allergen) and can include: [1]

- Runny nose and nasal congestion
- Watery or itchy eyes
- Sneezing
- Cough
- Itchy nose, roof of mouth or throat
- Sinus pressure and facial pain
- Swollen, blue-colored skin under the eyes (allergic shiners)
- Decreased sense of smell or taste

[1] http://www.mayoclinic.com/health/hay-fever

Honey is required in this remedy,

because it is believed that you will build a tolerance to bee pollen that exists in unfiltered honey. The ACV is believed to be the anti-inflammatory component.

Drink: Mix 2 T of apple cider vinegar and 2 T of honey in a glass of water three times a day preferably after each meal.

71) Head Lice

Prep Time: 10 min
Application Time: as desired

Ingredients:
1 C Apple Cider Vinegar+ enough water (bathing)
1 C Apple Cider Vinegar + 8 oz mineral oil
Nit comb
Shower cap

Directions:
To get rid of head lice try the following methods:

Bath: Add a cup of Apple Cider Vinegar to a quart of water and rinse your hair. Use a nit comb to search for lice. Repeat daily until the lice are gone.

Overnight Cap: Mix one cup of Apple Cider Vinegar to 8 oz of mineral oil. Drench your hair and scalp with this mixture, massaging through the hair. Cover your hair and scalp with the shower cap. Leave on overnight. Wash your hair the next morning with regular shampoo. Use nit comb to remove the lice and nits.

All bedding, clothing and potentially infected materials and surfaces must be washed well or the lice will easily return.

72) Headaches

Prep Time: 5-10 min
Application Time: as desired

Ingredients:
1 C Apple Cider Vinegar
1 C water
Vessel
Towel

Directions:
Apple cider vinegar when taken with honey can give relief from headaches.

During the headache attack, mix equal parts of apple cider vinegar and water in a round vessel and boil it on the stove.

Place the vessel at any place comfortable for you to inhale the fumes. Cover your face with a light towel and inhale the fumes coming from the mixture for a few minutes.

73) Hearing Disorders

Prep Time: 5 min
Application Time: 5 min

Ingredients:
2 T apple cider vinegar
8 oz distilled water

Directions:
Mix two tablespoons of apple cider vinegar into a glass of water and consume this three times a day. Apply diluted apple cider vinegar drops into the ear to help dissolve foreign matter.

Apple cider vinegar also kills bacteria, so it can help reduce the symptoms of minor infections.

74) Heart Disease

Prep Time: 5 min
Application Time: 5 min

Ingredients:
2T apple cider vinegar
8 oz distilled water

Directions:
Apple cider vinegar is a normalizing agent that can keep a check on both blood pressure and cholesterol levels. Acetic acid, a primary component in ACV, is the helpful ingredient in this situation

Drink: 2 T of Apple Cider Vinegar up to three times a day mixed with a glass of water after meals.

75) Heartburn

Prep Time: 5 min
Application Time: 5 min

Ingredients:
2 T apple cider vinegar
8 oz distilled water

Directions:
Heartburn often occurs after consuming food or beverages. It causes a pain in the chest and throat. This is due to improper functioning of the digestive system and imbalance of acid in the stomach. Apple Cider Vinegar consumed after meals is a good treatment for heartburn and also a prevention to this disease. For this, mix two tablespoons of Apple Cider Vinegar in a glass of a water and have it three times a day after meals.

"I recently saw a rather well thought out test of this remedy on the TV show Food Detectives. It seemed to work rather well, and the explanation was interesting. The heartburn is caused by acidic gases and liquid getting up into the esophagus, irritating the lining of the esophagus. The vinegar seems to trigger the sphincter like muscle at the lower end of the esophagus, causing it to tighten up and stop the 'leakage'."

http://voices.washingtonpost.com/checkup/2008/11/the_cide

r_vinegar_heartburn_cu.html

Apple cider vinegar consumed after meals is a good treatment for heartburn.

Drink: 2 T of apple cider vinegar in a glass of a water up to t h r e e times a day after meals

76) Heat Exhaustion

Prep Time: 5 min
Application Time: 5 min

Ingredients:
1 T apple cider vinegar
8 oz distilled water

Directions:
Exposure to sun for long periods or some activities in high heat makes the body lose water and electrolytes to cause heat exhaustion.

First symptoms include dryness of mouth and throat, tiredness and weakness, dizziness and even fainting. Continuing symptoms include nausea, profuse sweating and vomiting, headache, and muscle cramps.

Drinking cool water can give some relief but the body needs electrolytes for quick recovery.

Drink: 1 T of apple cider vinegar in a glass of water. Rehydrate with more water as necessary.

77) Heavy Metal Poisoning

Prep Time: 5 min
Application Time: 5 min

Ingredients:
2 T apple cider vinegar
8 oz distilled water

Directions:
Apple cider vinegar has been called the 'natural chelator.'

Organic apple cider vinegar has many vitamins, minerals and trace minerals that help with detoxifying the body.

Drink: Dilute apple cider vinegar, 2 T in a glass of water, three times a day.

78) Hemorrhoids

Prep Time: 5-10 min
Application Time: 4 to 7 min

Ingredients:
2 T Apple Cider Vinegar+ 8 oz water (drinking)
1 oz apple cider vinegar+ cotton ball (applying)

Directions:
Symptoms of hemorrhoids may include itching in the rectum area, and swelling and bleeding during bowel movements that cause rectal pain. Apple cider vinegar provides good, natural assistance for both internal and external hemorrhoids.

Apply: For treating external hemorrhoids, soak a cotton ball in vinegar and apply directly to the hemorrhoid

Drink: For internal treatment, drink two tablespoons of Apple Cider Vinegar mixed with a glass of water three times a day.

79) Hepatitis Support

Prep Time: 5 min
Application Time: 5 min

Ingredients:
2 T apple cider vinegar
8 oz distilled water

Directions:
Hepatitis damages and inflames liver cells. Apple Cider Vinegar contains malic and acetic acids that are considered helpful against viral diseases. ACV is anti-viral, anti-bacterial and anti-fungal.

Drink: 2 T of apple cider vinegar with a glass of water, three times a day.

80) Herpes

Prep Time: 5- 10 min
Application Time: 3 to 6 min

Ingredients:
1 T Apple Cider Vinegar
1 C water
Cotton ball

Directions:
Soak a cotton ball in apple cider vinegar and gently wipe lesions three to four times a day. The ACV acids will cause a burning feeling. When the burning is too strong, dilute the ACV with water to the strongest ACV strength tolerable. Herpes outbreaks can clear up in two to three days for simple blisters caught early.   Itching and irritation is greatly reduced.

81) Hiatal Hernia

Prep Time: 5 min
Application Time: 5 min

Ingredients:
2 T apple cider vinegar
8 oz distilled water

Directions:
Symptoms of Hiatal Hernia include heartburn, difficulty in swallowing, chest pain, and shortness of breath. Hiatal hernia symptoms can be treated with apple cider vinegar.

Mix two tablespoons of apple cider vinegar in a glass of water.

Drink this three times a day *after* meals.

82) Hiccups

Prep Time: 5 min
Application Time: 10 min

Ingredients:
1oz.apple cider vinegar
6 oz distilled water

Directions:
Pour a shot of apple cider vinegar.

Drink the shot.

Drink the water.

This is one of the oldest and easiest remedies for hiccups.

83) High Blood Pressure

Prep Time: 5 min
Application Time: 5 min

Ingredients:
1 T apple cider vinegar
8 oz distilled water

Directions:
Apple Cider Vinegar can help maintain a regular blood pressure, when consumed on a daily basis.

A 2006 study using ACV on mice and rats was able to help regulate blood pressure and lower cholesterol.

Dilute a tablespoon of apple cider vinegar in a glass of water and drink it three times a day.

84) High Cholesterol

Prep Time: 5 min
Application Time: 5 min

Ingredients:
1 T-2 T apple cider vinegar
8 oz distilled water

Directions:
It is believed that apple cider vinegar reduces cholesterol levels, because pectin prevents dietary cholesterol from being absorbed.

Mix one tablespoon of apple c ider v inegar in 8 Oz water and drink this three times a day with meals.

After 3 days, increase the amount of vinegar to two tablespoons.

85) Hives

Prep Time: 5-10 min
Application Time: 5-10 min

Ingredients:
1 oz Apple Cider Vinegar
2 oz water
Cotton ball

Directions:
Apple Cider Vinegar gives relief from the itching associated with hives. Mix one part Apple Cider Vinegar with two parts of water and apply on the affected area. When hives are on a larger section of the body, put the mixture in a spray bottle. Spray it on the affected area after having a bath.

86) Hot Flashes

Prep Time: 5 min
Application Time: 5 min

Ingredients:
2 T apple cider vinegar
8 oz distilled water

Directions:
To treat hot flashes, drink two tablespoons of Apple Cider Vinegar mixed with a glass of water every morning. This mixture can be taken up to three times a day. It is effective in reducing and controlling hot flashes of all kind including those in women during menopause.

http://www.earthclinic.com/CURES/hot_flashes.html

87) Hyperthyroidism

Prep Time: 5 min
Application Time: 5 min

Ingredients:
2 T apple cider vinegar
8 oz distilled water

Directions:
Hyperthyroidism causes low bone density. Apple Cider Vinegar contains minerals like manganese, calcium, magnesium, silicon and iron. All these help in developing bone mass and make the bones stronger. Take shots of Apple Cider Vinegar three times a day to help prevent problems related to Hyperthyroidism. For this, mix two tablespoons of vinegar to a glass of water.

88) Impetigo

Prep Time: 5-10 min
Application Time: 5 min

Ingredients:
1 oz Apple Cider Vinegar
4 oz water
Cotton ball

Directions:
Apple Cider Vinegar is an excellent therapy for Impetigo. Mix one part of Apple Cider Vinegar to four parts of water and apply it to the infected area 3-4 times daily.

89) Inflammation

Prep Time: 5-10 min
Application Time: as desired

Ingredients:

1 C Apple Cider Vinegar+ enough water (bathing)

1 T apple cider vinegar+1 C water+ cotton ball (applying)

2 T Apple Cider Vinegar+ 8 oz distilled water (drinking)

Directions:

The anti-inflammatory properties of Apple Cider Vinegar work for both external and internal inflammation.

Bath: For inflammation on skin caused by sunburn, add a cup of Apple Cider Vinegar in a bucket of water and have a bath with this mixture

Apply: Mix a tablespoon of vinegar to a cup of water and apply directly on the affected area.

Drink: For internal inflammation, mix two tablespoons of Apple Cider Vinegar with a glass of water and drink it three times a day during meals. It can also be added to salads.

90) Insect bites

Ingredients:
1 T Apple Cider Vinegar
1 C water
Cotton ball

Directions:
To treat insect bites, mix a tablespoon of Apple Cider Vinegar with a cup of water and apply on the bite with soft cotton ball. It has anti-inflammatory properties that will sooth the bite. It can stop the itching, bring relief from pain and reduce swelling.

91) Insomnia

Prep Time: 5 min
Application Time: 5 min

Ingredients:
2 t. apple cider vinegar
8 oz distilled water

Directions:
Apple Cider Vinegar and honey treatments can be a boon for many suffering from insomnia. Mix two teaspoons of Apple Cider Vinegar and equal quantity of honey in a glass of water. Drink this before going to bed. You can also keep another glass ready at your bedside and sip it, in case you wake up during the night.

92) Irregular Heartbeat

Prep Time: 5 min
Application Time: 5 min

Ingredients:
2 T apple cider vinegar
8 oz distilled water

Directions:

High potassium content of Apple Cider Vinegar is efficient in treating irregular heartbeats. Two tablespoons of Apple Cider Vinegar can either be taken diluted in a glass of water three times a day or can be used in salads.

93) Irritable Bowel Syndrome

Prep Time: 5 min
Application Time: 5 min

Ingredients:
2 T apple cider vinegar
8 oz distilled water

Directions:
Irritable bowel syndrome, also known as IBS, is intolerance against intestinal movements, spasm pain, gas, and bloating. Drinking two tablespoons of Apple Cider Vinegar with a glass of water three times a day is a simple, but very effective remedy for IBS.

94) Itching

Prep Time: 5-10 min
Application Time: 5-15 min

Ingredients:
1 oz Apple Cider Vinegar
4 oz water
Cotton ball

Directions:
Itching can be an outcome of various reasons such as- exposure to chemicals, dirt, sun, insect bites or stings, chicken pox, parasites, weather changes, allergies etc. Apple Cider Vinegar is useful in almost all types of itching. Mix one part of Apple Cider Vinegar with 4 parts of water and apply on the affected area with a cotton ball at regular intervals throughout the day.

95) Itchy Bottom Syndrome

Prep Time: 5-15 min
Application Time: as desired

Ingredients:
1 oz Apple Cider Vinegar+ 1 oz water
Cotton pad
Surgical bandage

Directions:
Soak a cotton pad in Apple Cider Vinegar and place it on the itching area. Direct application of Apple Cider Vinegar can give a great burning sensation. If you cannot bear it, mix equal parts of Apple Cider Vinegar and water and then apply on the affected area. You can also soak a cotton pad in the solution and keep it overnight by adhering with hospital tape or bandages. Full strength ACV has been reported to burn highly sensitive skin in some people.

96) Jelly Fish Stings

Prep Time: 5 min
Application Time: 10 to 20 min

Ingredients:
1 oz Apple Cider Vinegar
Cotton pad

Directions:
The sting of the large box jellyfish is deadly. Sometimes the tentacles are left inside the body where it strikes. It continues to release poison. Apple Cider Vinegar, when applied on the bite area, has stopped the venom release. Apple Cider Vinegar can be seen in the first aid kit of lifeguards for rapid treatment.

97) Jock Itch

Prep Time: 5-10 min
Application Time: 10 min

Ingredients:
1 Apple Cider Vinegar
1 C water
Cotton pad

Directions:
Jock itch can be treated by applying diluted Apple Cider Vinegar on the affected area. Dilute a teaspoon of Apple Cider Vinegar in a cup of water. Apply to the infected area. Leave for 10 minutes and then remove. Repeat 3-4 times daily especially before going to bed.

98) Joint Aches

Prep Time: 10 min
Application Time: as desired

Ingredients:
2 T Apple cider vinegar+ 8 oz water (drinking)
2 T Apple cider vinegar+ 1 T mineral oil (massage)
1 C Apple cider vinegar+ enough water (soaking)

Directions:
Apple Cider Vinegar is rich in minerals like magnesium, phosphorus, calcium and potassium. When a deficiency of these minerals occurs in the body, joint pains can appear with increasing severity. People who suffer from joint pains are often found to be a victim of indigestion that leads to improper nutrient absorption from the food they eat.

Apple Cider Vinegar is also a very good digestive aide. Some experts believe that joint pains are a result of toxins that accumulate in the joints. Pectin in apple cider vinegar helps to absorb toxins and the alkalizing effect of ACV helps in detoxifying the whole system.

Drink: Consume two tablespoons of Apple Cider Vinegar mixed in a glass of water three times a day.

Apply: It can also be applied on the joint to get quick relief from pain. For this, mix two tablespoons apple cider vinegar with one tablespoon of mineral oil and massage into the joints.

Soak: For ankle and wrist pain, you can soak the area in one cup of apple cider vinegar mixed with about half bucket of water.

99) Kidney Disease Support

Prep Time: 5 min
Application Time: 5 min

Ingredients:
2 T apple cider vinegar
8 oz distilled water

Directions:
Most of the kidney and urinary tract infections can be treated by including apple cider vinegar in the diet. ACV helps to reduce inflammation and alkalize the body. ACV should be considered a high potassium food that must be avoided by people with kidney failure or serious kidney disease.

Drink two tablespoons of apple cider vinegar with a glass of water three times a day to flush out toxins and harmful bacteria

100) Kidney stones

Prep Time: 5 min
Application Time: 5 min

Ingredients:
6-8 t. apple cider vinegar
24 oz distilled water

Directions:
Mix 6 -8 teaspoons Apple Cider Vinegar in 3 quarts of purified water. Drink this throughout the day instead of plain water. Many people found relief from pain within 2 days. This can also reduce the size of the stones and can sometimes cause stones to disappear completely.

101) Toe Fungus

Prep Time: 10 min
Application Time: as desired

Ingredients:
2 T Apple cider vinegar+ 8 oz water (drinking)
2 T Apple cider vinegar+ 1 T water (massage)
1 C Apple cider vinegar+ enough water (soaking)

Directions:
About once per week file the nail down as thin as possible without breaking through it. Be careful not to cut the skin around it either. Drink Apple Cider Vinegar daily to help alkalize your system and be sure to soak or massage the diluted Apple Cider Vinegar into the nail and toe throughout the day.

Drink: Consume two tablespoons of Apple Cider Vinegar mixed in a glass of water three times a day.

Apply: Apply the ACV on the toenail and the toe three times per day.

Soak: Your toe and foot in one cup of Apple Cider Vinegar mixed with about 3 cups of water for soaking.

102) Cleaning Agents

Prep Time: 10 min
Application Time: as desired

Ingredients:

1 part Apple Cider Vinegar : 1 part water
(General cleaner/Glass/Mirrors)
Full strength – Spot Remover

Directions:

ACV is an outstanding cleaner!
Use the general cleaner strength in spray bottles and washcloths to clean

Windows
Mirrors
Kitchen and bath countertops

Cook tops
Wipe stain marks off walls

Add full strength to clean
Laundry stains

Carpet stains (spot test)
Trashcans
Cleaning toilet stains

103) Weight Loss

High quality Apple Cider Vinegar is the best addition you can put into any diet or weight loss program. Apple Cider Vinegar actually helps your body get rid of annoying hunger cravings. By taking Apple Cider Vinegar 15 minutes before each meal you will not be as hungry. You will find it easier to stop eating. Weight loss and diabetes sugar control are two of the few scientifically studied areas in apple cider vinegar.

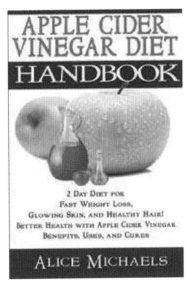

Are you trying to control hunger and lose weight?
I recommend my book on the Apple Cider Vinegar diet:

Apple Cider Vinegar DIET Handbook
by Alice Michaels

Control Hunger

You can gain numerous benefits by supplementing with apple cider vinegar. This is because, organic, freshly crushed, Apple Cider Vinegar has the ability to increase metabolism and help regulate glucose digestion.

Regulating sugar digestion helps minimize blood glucose spikes that create a cycle of hunger. That alone made ACV worth trying to use as a diet aide. So....I did!

When I first became interested in apple cider vinegar, I wanted to take off a few extra pounds that I hoped would jump-start an exercise program. My motivation was not very high to get in shape, but that quickly changed with the ACV.

Start With Less

Why would I use only one to two teaspoons, when one to two Tablespoons would do the trick?

One Tablespoon is actually 3 times what was originally recommended, although it has now become a standard in many ACV weight loss drinks. I recommend you start with a smaller amount and then try increasing the ACV.

The first time I used ACV was as an addition to a diet I had already been on for weeks. It appeared I plateaued. I dropped 8 pounds within the following two weeks. The ACV got me back on track quickly. I use Bragg's which I highly recommend.

104) Get the Glow of Healthier Skin

Apple cider vinegar benefits also include healthier skin.

Help your skin from the inside by drinking the ACV drink up to 3 times each day. This improves your overall health by keeping the body alkaline and above all leaving your skin aglow.

From the outside, use the Rosemary Skin Tonic recipe above. Apple cider vinegar has enzymes as well as ascetic acid that can remove skin surface fatty deposits and reduce problem skin by regulating the pH.

Apple cider vinegar is also an antibacterial. Many people discover a reduction in uneven skin color, dryness and acne once the pH is balanced.

By maintaining the proper pH balance of your skin, you help to avoid acne and other skin infections and thus maintain a healthy skin.

See: ACV Healthy Glow Rosemary Skin Tonic under RECIPES

105) Helps to Regulate Blood Pressure

Regulating blood pressure is just one in the long list of benefits of ACV. This is made possible because of the vinegars acetic acid composition, which, as shown in a study conducted in 2001, is known to be relevant in lowering blood pressure. ACV breaks down mucous and body fat to help create greater arterial integrity that aids in lowering blood pressure.

106) Topical Bath Astringent & Detox

One of the best plus factors of apple cider vinegar is that it is helpful in alleviating most types of skin problems. The composition of apple cider has the capacity to absorb excess oil from the skin, help balance the pH levels and to kill bacteria. This natural ingredient can be used as a sort of topical astringent for any type of skin that is experiencing problems.

Simple Skin Application: A mixture of one part vinegar and three parts water can be applied to the skin using a cotton swab and be applied to the skin three times a day for ten minutes each.

Bath Detox: Another method would be to add a cup of ACV to a cup of salt in hot bath in order to help release the toxins from the skin.

107) Natural anti-aging medicine

As medicine progressed, people have become obsessed with the idea of making themselves younger than their actual age. This magic is done with the help of powerful supplements available in the market that all promise the reduction of wrinkles as well as the other signs of aging.

"An apple cider vinegar benefit is that it is a simple do-it-yourself, anti-wrinkle skin toner solution that proves to be rather effective as anti-aging with the bonus of being a natural tonic."

See: Recipes Skin Tonic and Facial Steamer

108) Gargle and Swish for Whiter Teeth

Each morning swish a little apple cider vinegar and water around your teeth to help remove stains. Then gargle with the remaining product and swallow.

ACV helps to kill bacteria in your gums and the mouth while whitening your teeth, so it is a helpful addition to your mouth care routine.

I love brushing with ACV, too, but the acid level is too much to leave on your teeth for a long time.

Make sure you brush your teeth as usual after you gargle.

109) Natural Hair Conditioner & Scalp Tonic

Apple cider vinegar is exceptional for strong, curly, wiry hair. For your hair, make a solution of ACV with water mixed in equal proportions. The shorter your hair means the less you will need, so mix up what you will need fresh each time.

I like to use a one-pint plastic bottle with a pointed tip. I have thick hair, so it is easy to squirt it on my hair and massage it to the scalp. You can dilute this to 50% of original. I do not get any burning with full strength, but that's me. Be sure to test it. There is no need to feel a burn on your scalp to get the benefits. Add enough water to find the strength that works best for you.

This is great as a scalp tonic especially for those who have less or thinning hair. Put it in a spray bottle and massage it onto the scalp. Be sure you know where you are spraying, because your bathroom will smell like vinegar when the mist is allowed elsewhere in the room. Leave this on your hair and scalp for a half hour before rinsing it off.

Reminder: Do you keep your water and ACV in the refrigerator as I do? Take out what you need the night before to let it warm. Apple Cider Vinegar serves as a natural hair conditioner. It helps nourish your hair leaving it with a shiny soft texture. The feeling afterward is very fresh and clean. Be sure to rinse with water one extra time. I like to use the tonic recipe above with rosemary sprigs. It freshens the scent just enough without leaving that overpowering ACV scent.

110) Get Rid of Skin tags

There seem to be hundreds of ways reported to get skin tags to fall off, but even so, not every method has worked well for everyone.

Here is the apple cider vinegar method that has great results without a lot of side effects of chemicals or the difficulties and embarrassment of using tying string.

- Day 1: Put undiluted ACV on a cotton ball. Put that onto the tag and then cover it with a bandage just before going to bed on.
- Day 2: Do the steps in Day 1 again. (Sensitive areas and sensitive skin may get itchy or red, so remove it and wait for the next day. Cover it with a bandage to protect it.)
- Do this for 1 week: By the end of the week, the tag will have turned gray to black and then will have fallen off.

Note: I use undiluted ACV, because my skin is not over sensitive to burning from the acetic acid. For those who are, first try a solution of 25% ACV + 75% water. Of course, results are not as quick, so decide what strength works best for your skin type.

Why Bragg's Organic Apple Cider Vinegar

Bragg's Organic Apple Cider Vinegar is consistently an outstanding product that has been scientifically tested.

The "mother" is always present and the product is never pasteurized.
This is the conclusion of the study:

CONCLUSION

These data indicate that daily vinegar consumption favorably influences fasting glucose concentrations in healthy adults and contribute important information to the growing evidence base supporting the antiglycemic effects of vinegar.

Vinegar is inexpensive, readily available, and a flavor enhancer. Although vinegar was taken as a drink prior to mealtime in the present study, vinegar can be incorporated into meals as a vinaigrette dressing on salads or vegetables or as a sandwich spread in the form of mustard, or it can simply be spritzed onto

foods. Note that commercial vinegar tablets do not contain adequate amounts of

acetic acid to induce an antiglycemic effect.

I take my Apple Cider Vinegar Drink up to three times daily. (See: recipe MyFavorite)
This book lists the many reasons why I find Apple Cider Vinegar so extremely beneficial to me and those I love.

I also purchase the smaller quart bottle unless the gallons are priced at a significant savings.
Although apple cider vinegar will last for years, especially when kept in the refrigerator, there is still an oxidation that takes place. My rule of thumb is to use my opened quart within 60 days of opening. That's easy to do, because I'll have an ounce a day or share it with someone, so it won't last a month.

Bragg's is now sold in grocery and health food stores. Watch out particularly for multiple quart or gallon sales that you would expect to save you money over a single quart price. They can be significantly higher and shipping still is tacked on at the end.

Apple Cider Vinegar Benefits & Disease

How ACV May Help Protect Against Some Cancers

Your body has an overall pH. That is the reference used to understand just how alkaline or acidic your body is. A state less than 7pH (the pH of water) is chemically known as Acidic. Seven pH is neutral and anything above it is Alkaline. Many diseases cannot thrive in an alkaline environment, but many people have a pH that is too acidic, allowing disease to find a home and create havoc. Small studies do show that apple cider vinegar can kill cancers and even slow down the development of cancer cells.

Organic, unfiltered, unpasteurized apple cider vinegar made from raw apples is much healthier than other types of vinegar because it has an alkalizing effect to the body.

Not All Vinegars Are the Same

White vinegar can be made from grains like corn and even fruits, like apples, but much of it is made from *petroleum*. When it does not say that white vinegar is made from grains, then assume it is not. Synthetic ethanol added to white vinegar is not considered a safe food product by the USFDA. Since synthetic ethanol use has not been challenged in court, the FDA allows it in our food supply.

Why would people think their food is healthy enough to heal them when they cannot trust simple products that have been on store shelves for decades?

I believe that is why a few good choices that improve the diet make astounding changes quickly.

Apple cider vinegar with the 'mother' is one of those products.

The alkalizing effect makes the body less acidic and more alkaline. A more alkaline body prevents many diseases from obtaining the proper environment to thrive. Other types of vinegars can make your body more acidic; this environment is a good environment to cause illness.

Tummy Troubles

Apple cider vinegar for tummy troubles has been a Godsend to me.

When I have occasional indigestion, I will put a tablespoonful of ACV in a measuring cup. Drink it and follow it with water.

When you have digestion problems such as diarrhea, this vinegar will help contain the problem. Supposedly, it is due to the antibiotic properties of ACV that eliminate bacterial infection in the stomach.

I do know the extra acid is helpful when I have overeaten or had improper foods that leave my stomach to do the job right.

People claim that ACV vinegar also contains pectin, which is very beneficial in soothing intestinal spasms.

Apple cider vinegar curbs many indigestion problems. Before you eat foods that you think may lead to stomach problems, sip this vinegar. Add one teaspoon of honey and one teaspoon of ACV to a warm glass of water. Drink 30 minutes before eating your meal.

Fight Cold and Cough

ACV combined with honey and water is one the best remedies for cold, cough and a sore throat. Mix one teaspoon of ACV, one teaspoon of honey and one teaspoon of warm water. You can also add some smashed ginger to the mixture to enhance its medicinal properties. Take this mixture three times a day. I use it to give me relief from cough and congestion, when the only other items I could turn to were drugs. There is a time for taking medications, but when something as simple as ACV can help clean me up and get me going, I'll be happy to use it.

Alleviate Infection Symptoms

Apple cider vinegar exhibits antiseptic properties and has helped in the fight against fungal and bacterial infections. Apple cider vinegar is beneficial when dealing with bladder infections, ear infections, candida and other infections. Drink a glass of warm water and ACV each night to alleviate the symptoms of bladder infections and candida. For ear infections, rinse the ear with diluted apple cider vinegar. Be careful putting anything in the ear canal. Even cotton swabs can puncture the eardrum. Many pharmacies now sell liquid delivery syringes specifically designed to minimize entry into the ear canal. Ask your pharmacists for information on these over the counter safety products.

Improve Bone Health

ACV is rich in potassium, calcium, magnesium and other essential minerals. This makes it very beneficial in maintain bone health. It is known to keep your bones strong and help prevent osteoporosis and other bone diseases. Drink the ACV drink a few times a day and watch joint pain eased.

Combat Diabetes

Here is great news for those living with diabetes who find carb-control and exercise not enough to lower sugar values. The acetic acid in apple cider vinegar reduces carbohydrate assimilation to a slower, more even level after eating food, so the blood sugar values do not spike as much. How much? Small studies have shown ACV can reduce sugar highs by as much as 20%(avg was 4% to 6%) and for many people that is enough to win the battle. For others it is a healthier road that minimizes sugar damage.

Apple cider vinegar is beneficial to diabetes patients and people with blood sugar problems in more than one way. It helps by slowing down the release of insulin and post meal glucose. Therefore, this vinegar has the ability to slow down sugar piling up in the blood stream.

Are you diabetic? Then you can easily try this effect by measuring your blood sugar frequently throughout the day a couple of hours before and after you have had the ACV drink.

I have diabetes II. I get tremendous benefit with Apple Cider Vinegar.

ACV is not a substitute for taking care of myself in larger ways, but there are simply times when I say yes to a special night out or a special goodie. Apple Cider Vinegar gives me that slight edge to let me say yes.

Of course, I watch my diet, but I still fall off the wagon from time to time. ACV helps me get around those difficult times when I would rather splurge. As long as I have been doing well with my diet, then a little extra here and there has been fine for me, especially with the addition of ACV in my diet.

I also exercise, but not as regularly as I used to. Aerobic exercise burns off extra sugar and helps to keep off those extra pounds. I know it is good to do, but fitting it into my schedule isn't easy. Apple cider vinegar is certainly not a replacement for exercise, but it is one extra important item in my arsenal that lets me live my life on my terms. The smallest changes in life can make the greatest impact.

In summary, ACV is a super product that helps to rid food cravings, and even out my sugar highs and lows. As great as it is, I would not consider ACV as the diabetes cure, but it is an outstanding tool that gives me an edge toward sugar control. Regular exercise and following an extra clean diet are major components to enjoying a healthy life.

Apple Cider Vinegar Side Effects

The negative side effects I read seem about seem to refer to the same, few medical stories. They are stories, because just as apple cider vinegar has received few multi-million dollar scientific, double-blind studies, so, too, is there no serious science backing up the nutritionists' assumptions.

This comes from the Mayo Health Clinic website:

> *"Apple cider vinegar is highly acidic. It may irritate your throat if you drink it often or in large amounts."*

> *"Apple cider vinegar may interact with certain supplements or drugs, including diuretics and insulin. This may contribute to low potassium levels."*

Apple cider vinegar contains acetic acid that is actually considered mild,, but so is the acid in citrus fruits, grapefruits

"Long-term risks associated with apple cider vinegar use include low blood potassium levels, diminished bone mineral density and a burning feeling in the throat from repeated ingestion." Apple cider vinegar is often not pasteurized or not filtered properly and may contain harmful bacteria. The acid level in vinegar is sufficient to keep out most bacteria.

Its acidic properties may also damage the digestive tract and esophagus, and also change tooth enamel. Reports show that apple cider vinegar can also lower bone density and potassium levels. Strong vinegar can cause skin irritations and even burning or scarring of the organs like the stomach and liver, especially if it is not properly diluted. Also, medical reports indicate that there is the potential for acid chemical burns from apple cider vinegar in pill form. Much caution should be used when drinking or using apple cider vinegar on the skin to remove age spots.

Read more:
 http://www.skincareguide.com/article/age-spots-removal-does-apple-cider-vinegar-really-work.html#ixzz2Tc91Alpb

Recipes

In all recipes, I use organic, unfiltered, unpasteurized, raw apple cider vinegar that has been refrigerated and not open longer than 60 days. Apple cider vinegar lasts for years, but the best and most mild flavor comes right after opening the bottle. My first choice is Bragg's Organic Apple Cider Vinegar. I have been using it for years and I trust the consistency.

Apple Cider Vinegar Drink Recipe I

Ingredients: :

1t. to 3t. Apple Cider Vinegar
8 oz   Warm water
1 T   Honey or Stevia to taste

Directions:

Mix the Ingredients: in a glass jar. I like to shake it for a minute until frothy. Normally drink this on an empty stomach, but some people get an irritated stomach for a short time afterward. Should that happen to you, try drinking an extra glass of water first. Recipes have varied from 1 teaspoon to 1 Tablespoon (=3 teaspoons).

The original recipes call for honey, because honey adds enzymes and vitamins that aide digestion. It is my personal choice not to eat honey. I prefer to sweeten foods with stevia.

Apple Cider Vinegar Drink Recipe II

Ingredients: :

1 T   Apple Cider Vinegar
6 oz Warm water
1 T   Blackstrap Molasses

Directions:

Add the Ingredients: to your mixing jar and shake for a minute until frothy. Add more water if you want and drink. I love blackstrap molasses, which already has a good assortment of vitamins and minerals, especially organic iron.

Apple Cider Vinegar Chaser (My Favorite)

Ingredients: :

1T   Apple Cider Vinegar

8 oz   COLD water

1 t   Fresh ginger root, minced(optional)

Directions:

Pour the apple cider vinegar into a small cup. Shoot it back into your throat as though you're drinking with the gals down at the rowdy pub. Keep the cold water chaser handy. Sip it until you've had your fill. Easy & done.

I like apple cider vinegar now and have no problem taking my next drink, as long as I make sure that I have everything this way:

1. Always drink from a fresh bottle that has not been opened more than a couple months. A bottle does not last in my house that long, but the flavor becomes too harsh when it sits too long.
2. Keep the ACV bottle in a cold refrigerator.
3. Drink filtered, cold water to make this all seem that much better for me.

To the sensitive skin types, be careful. Apple cider vinegar is very acidic. There have been a few reports that it has burned the mouth or throat and damaged tooth enamel when left on the teeth in full strength for too long.

I recommend rinsing immediately with the cold water and drinking an equivalent amount of water to the vinegar to dilute it.

I have never had a problem with burning, even after drinking it full strength or putting it on my skin full strength. We are not all built the same, so your experience may be different. Test by diluting the full strength vinegar by adding an equal amount of water first. Talk with your health professional to see what optimum is for you should you have concerns.

Apple Cider Vinegar Gargle

Ingredients: :

¼ c Apple Cider Vinegar

¼ c Water

This 50/50 solution of ACV and water helps kill germs in the throat and mouth, so it is great for that sore throat and mouth pain caused by germs.

Do you have extremely sensitive mouth and throat areas?   Then double the water to reduce the acid strength first.   Rinse your mouth afterwards to remove ACV from your teeth.

ACV Healthy Glow Rosemary Skin Tonic

8 oz   Apple Cider Vinegar
2   Rosemary, fresh herb, dried sprigs
2 T   Witch Hazel Extract, optional
2 T   Organic Aloe Vera Juice
2 T   Vegetable Glycerin

Add the apple cider vinegar and rosemary together into a clear bottle that is capped and placed in the sun for a day or two.

Add the Witch Hazel Extract and Vegetable Glycerin

Added liquids change the pH so I choose to keep this refrigerated for up to a week.

You can omit the Witch Hazel, but it is a favorite I learned from my mother.

ACV Facial Skin Steamer

2 oz   Apple Cider Vinegar

1 qt Water

1 sprig   Fresh Rosemary, optional

Heat the 2 oz of apple cider vinegar with the 1 quart of water until a gentle steam appears.

Place your face into the steam and cover your head trapping the steam with a towel.

This type of facial steaming was popular in the 1950's and 1960's. It helps to open and clean out pores. Of course, be careful not to create a steam burn by trapping too much steam at one time.

You can do this over the stove, but it's risky.

I absolutely love a home facial steamer. I've used the steamer below for years. It's easy to use.

Add water. Turn on. Steam. You feel so fresh after an Apple Cider Vinegar facial steam.

Simple Salad Dressing

½ c. Apple Cider Vinegar

2 T Freshly Squeezed Lemon Juice

¼ t. Dried Parsley

¼ t. Dried Basil

1 T Clover Honey or Stevia to taste

½ c. Extra Virgin Olive Oil

¼ t. Sea Salt

¼ t. Freshly Ground Pepper

Add Ingredients: into a jar.

Shake until well mixed.

Refrigerate until chilled.

Shake before serving.

Serve over greens or sliced tomatoes and cucumbers.

Simplest Salad Dressing

If you were to look in my refrigerator, you would always find enough food to feed the neighborhood. That means the dressing bottles are partly full and never sure which direction they should go.

Take two of your favorites and top a salad with a little of each.
Then pour on a little apple cider vinegar.
Add enough for each person to have one to two teaspoons.
Toss the salad & Serve.

What a great way to get a serving of apple cider vinegar into the diet! Make the salad extra tasty with some almonds and toasted hazelnuts for crunch. Once you find two or three combinations that make an easy-to-assemble salad flavorful, you will find it easier to make those other better diet choices a regular part of the day.

Questions & Answers

Does Apple Cider Vinegar Go Bad?

Each bottle has a 'use by' date that I like to follow, but just as I was about to send this book to print, I found a bottle in the back of a storage refrigerator. This bottle was opened and probably passed the use by date, but the marking was worn off and I could not tell. The bottle was chilled for months. Even so, the color was darker than my fresh bottle and it appeared to be clearer.

When I tried a tablespoon that was not diluted, the apple cider vinegar was very strong, almost harsh. I opened my fresh bottle and did the same thing, but the flavor was smooth and easy to take. Older apple cider vinegar, even refrigerated very cold for months, may be fine, but the flavor can make it difficult to take.

Why Use Cold Water and Cold ACV?

I prefer cold water, especially when regulating weight. Eight ounces of cold water uses an additional 100 calories to warm up. Cold reduces the ability to taste a food, too. Cold foods, such as ice cream, need extra sweetener and more of most flavorings so the desired tastes come through the cold.

There is a potential downside to drinking very cold (and very hot) liquids. The shock to your teeth can cause small cracks. When you drink an iced drink, use a straw to get the cold liquid past your teeth.

.

Conclusion

There are hundreds of apple cider vinegar benefits reported over 1000's of years. I included my favorites with easy information on how you can benefit yourself from this amazing product, Apple Cider Vinegar.

To exploit the full vinegar benefits, be sure to use raw, organic, unfiltered and unpasteurized vinegar. This type of apple cider vinegar has 'mother of vinegar' content and contains the highest number of nutrients, enzymes and helpful bacteria. This cobweb-like substance may look strange but it is your key to getting the many apple cider vinegar benefits waiting for you.

You can easily get apple cider vinegar into your diet. Combine a few teaspoons with a glass of water and drink before you have your meal. See the recipes above.

Include ACV into your food, especially in salad dressings. You can buy apple cider vinegar as a digestive and blood sugar support supplement, but it is a great addition to your daily diet in so many recipes.

There are different brands of apple cider vinegar. I trust Bragg's, because I have used it for years and the product remains consistent and good. It is organic, not filtered, not pasteurized, has no synthetic additives. Today I buy it from local grocery stores that offer nice sales from time to time.

I love apple cider vinegar even as a cold drink, the colder the better for me. Bottled apple cider vinegar with the mother is still best. During road trips or long weekends away from my kitchen, I now buy ACV bottled drinks or create ACV drinks myself at home and store in a cooler for travel.

Special Thanks to YOU!

Obtain Your FREE copy of my book "Fat Loss Booster Tips – Get a Boost

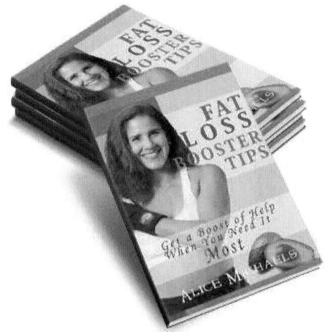

of Help When You Need it Most"

Did you get your FREE copy of my book? Just go to this link on the internet and you will get all the extras as my gift. ($14.95 value)

Fat Loss Booster Tips – Get a Boost of Help When You Need it Most

http://www.m8u.org/HealthyBonus/